In what ways can yoga be done

Yoga is good for health

Q. BANKS

Table of Contents

Introduction

Yoga is a physical, mental, and otherworldly practice that began in old India. It includes a progression of stances, breathing activities, and contemplation methods that advance physical and mental prosperity.

The actual stances, or asanas, help to further develop adaptability, strength, equilibrium, and coordination. The breathing activities, or pranayama, help to quiet the brain, diminish pressure, and increment oxygen stream to the body. Reflection strategies, or dhyana, help to concentrate the psyche and work on mental clearness.

Yoga is frequently polished for its medical advantages, like lessening pressure and uneasiness, working on cardiovascular wellbeing, and easing persistent agony. It is likewise utilized as an otherworldly work on, assisting specialists with interfacing with a higher power or internal identity.

There are various kinds of yoga, including Hatha, Vinyasa, Ashtanga, Bikram, and Kundalini, among others. Each type underlines various parts of the training and might be more qualified to various people in view of their objectives and capacities.

Hatha Yoga

Hatha Yoga is a traditional style of yoga that started in old India. It is the most generally drilled style of yoga and is the underpinning of numerous different styles of yoga. Hatha Yoga centers around actual stances, known as asanas, and breathing strategies, known as pranayama, determined to advance actual wellbeing and mental prosperity.

"Hatha" is a Sanskrit word that signifies "power" or "exertion". In Hatha Yoga, the accentuation is on creating strength and adaptability in the body, as well as developing a profound consciousness of the breath and the brain.

The act of Hatha Yoga includes a mix of actual stances, breathing procedures, and reflection. The actual stances, or asanas, are intended to extend and reinforce the muscles, further develop adaptability, and increment course all through the body. The breathing strategies, or pranayama, are utilized to quiet the psyche, lessen pressure, and increment energy levels. Contemplation is utilized to assist with calming the brain and foster a more profound feeling of mindfulness and internal harmony.

One of the vital standards of Hatha Yoga is the idea of "stirha" and "sukha", and that signifies "consistent" and "agreeable" individually. In Hatha Yoga, the stances are intended to be testing, yet reachable, permitting the specialist to track down a harmony among exertion and straightforwardness. The objective is to discover a feeling of solace and straightforwardness in each stance, while as yet keeping a consistent and centered mind.

One more significant standard of Hatha Yoga is the idea of "prana", which alludes to the existence force energy that moves through the body. The act of pranayama is intended to help balance and direct the progression of prana, which can assist with working on generally wellbeing and prosperity.

Hatha Yoga can be polished by individuals of any age and capacities, as the stances can be altered to suit individual necessities and impediments. It is an extraordinary style of yoga for fledglings, as it gives a strong groundwork to other yoga styles. Nonetheless, even experienced specialists can profit from the act of Hatha Yoga, as it gives a chance to extend their attention to the body, breath, and brain.

In a run of the mill Hatha Yoga class, you can hope to travel through a progression of actual stances, holding each posture for a few breaths. The stances can go from straightforward stretches to more complicated adjusting postures and reversals. The class may likewise incorporate pranayama procedures and contemplation, which can assist with quieting the psyche and extend the training.

One of the vital advantages of rehearsing Hatha Yoga is worked on actual wellbeing. The stances can assist with further developing adaptability, strength, equilibrium, and coordination, as well as increment course and work on in general cardiovascular

wellbeing. Normal practice can likewise assist with easing side effects of persistent agony, like back torment and joint inflammation.

Notwithstanding the actual advantages, Hatha Yoga can likewise assist with working on psychological well-being and prosperity. The act of pranayama and reflection can assist with decreasing pressure and uneasiness, further develop fixation and concentration, and advance sensations of serenity and inward harmony. Standard practice can likewise assist with further developing rest and increment energy levels.

Generally, Hatha Yoga is a flexible and open style of yoga that can be polished by anybody, no matter what their age or capacity. It gives a chance to foster strength, adaptability, and inward mindfulness, as well as advance by and large wellbeing and prosperity. With ordinary practice, Hatha Yoga can assist with working on actual wellbeing, mental clearness, and profound prosperity, prompting a more adjusted and satisfying life.

Vinyasa Yoga

Vinyasa Yoga is a dynamic and streaming style of yoga that started in India. It is a famous style of yoga in the Western world, and is known for its accentuation on smooth motions, synchronized breath, and imaginative sequencing of stances. In Vinyasa Yoga, the asanas, or stances, are connected together in a succession, with every development facilitated with a particular breathe in or breathe out of the breath.

"Vinyasa" comes from the Sanskrit expression "nyasa", and that signifies "to place", and "vi", and that signifies "in an extraordinary way". In Vinyasa Yoga, the stances are set in a particular grouping that is intended to make a streaming and dynamic practice. The act of Vinyasa Yoga is many times portrayed as a moving contemplation, as the persistent development and centered breath help to quiet the brain and extend familiarity with the body and breath.

One of the vital standards of Vinyasa Yoga is the idea of "ujjayi" breath, and that signifies "triumphant breath". This is a particular kind of breathing that is utilized in Vinyasa Yoga to assist with directing the breath and quiet the psyche. The ujjayi breath is described by a delicate, discernible sound that is made by choking the muscles toward the rear of the throat. This sort of breathing assists with making a feeling of inner intensity and concentration, which can assist with developing the training.

One more significant standard of Vinyasa Yoga is the idea of "vinyasa krama", and that signifies "bit by bit movement". In Vinyasa Yoga, the stances are connected together in a particular grouping, with every development facilitated with a particular breathe in or breathe out of the breath. This assists with making a feeling of smoothness and stream in the training, while likewise assisting with developing fortitude and perseverance.

In a normal Vinyasa Yoga class, you can hope to travel through a progression of actual stances, holding each posture for a few breaths prior to changing into the following posture. The class may likewise incorporate pranayama procedures and contemplation, which can assist with extending the training and advance a feeling of tranquility and unwinding.

One of the vital advantages of rehearsing Vinyasa Yoga is worked on actual wellbeing. The persistent development and dynamic sequencing of stances can assist with further developing adaptability, strength, balance, and cardiovascular wellbeing. Normal practice can likewise assist with mitigating side effects of constant torment, like back agony and joint inflammation.

Notwithstanding the actual advantages, Vinyasa Yoga can likewise assist with working on emotional well-being and prosperity. The act of ujjayi breath and contemplation can assist with diminishing pressure and tension, further develop fixation and concentration, and advance sensations of tranquility and inward harmony. Normal practice can likewise assist with further developing rest and increment energy levels.

In general, Vinyasa Yoga is a difficult and dynamic style of yoga that is open to individuals of any age and capacities. It gives a valuable chance to foster strength, adaptability, and internal mindfulness, as well as advance generally speaking wellbeing and prosperity. With normal practice, Vinyasa Yoga can assist with working on actual wellbeing, mental clearness, and profound prosperity, prompting a more adjusted and satisfying life.

Ashtanga Yoga

Ashtanga Yoga is a dynamic and truly requesting style of yoga that was created by Sri K. Pattabhi Jois in the twentieth hundred years. A customary type of yoga follows a set grouping of stances, or asanas, and is described by serious areas of strength for an on the breath, interior intensity, and streaming development.

The expression "Ashtanga" signifies "eight appendages", and alludes to the eight appendages of yoga as framed in the antiquated text, the Yoga Sutras of Patanjali. These appendages incorporate moral standards, actual stances, breath control, sense withdrawal, fixation, contemplation, and edification. Ashtanga Yoga centers basically around the actual stances, or asanas, for of accomplishing the higher conditions of cognizance depicted in the Yoga Sutras.

The act of Ashtanga Yoga is partitioned into six series of stances, every one of which is further developed than the last. The principal series, known as the Essential Series, is the underpinning of the training and is intended to cleanse the body and develop fortitude and adaptability. Every series starts with a set grouping of sun greetings, trailed by a succession of standing stances, situated stances, backbends, and reversals.

One of the critical standards of Ashtanga Yoga is the idea of vinyasa, which alludes to the synchronization of breath and development. In Ashtanga Yoga, every development is facilitated with either a breathe in or a breathe out of the breath, making a streaming and dynamic practice. The breath is likewise utilized for the purpose of creating inward intensity, which assists with purging the body and extend the training.

One more significant rule of Ashtanga Yoga is the idea of drishti, and that signifies "look" or "concentration". Each stance in the training has a particular drishti, or place of concentration, which assists with coordinating the energy and consideration of the professional. By centering the look, the brain can turn out to be more engaged and thought, which can assist with developing the training and advance a feeling of inward quiet and tranquility.

Ashtanga Yoga is a difficult and truly requesting practice, and isn't suggested for fledglings or those with wounds or wellbeing concerns. In any case, with standard practice and commitment, Ashtanga Yoga can assist with developing fortitude, adaptability, and perseverance, as well as advance mental clearness and profound prosperity.

One of the critical advantages of rehearsing Ashtanga Yoga is worked on actual wellbeing. The persistent development and dynamic sequencing of stances can assist with further developing adaptability, strength, balance, and cardiovascular wellbeing. Customary practice can likewise assist with mitigating side effects of constant agony, like back torment and joint pain.

Notwithstanding the actual advantages, Ashtanga Yoga can likewise assist with working on emotional well-being and prosperity. The act of vinyasa and drishti can assist with lessening pressure and uneasiness, further develop fixation and concentration, and advance sensations of smoothness and inward harmony. Standard practice can likewise assist with further developing rest and increment energy levels.

Generally, Ashtanga Yoga is a difficult and dynamic style of yoga that is grounded in custom and zeroed in on physical and mental cleaning. It gives a potential chance to foster strength, adaptability, and inward mindfulness, as well as advance in general wellbeing and prosperity. With customary practice, Ashtanga Yoga can assist with working on actual wellbeing, mental lucidity, and close to home prosperity, prompting a more adjusted and satisfying life.

Bikram Yoga

Bikram Yoga, otherwise called hot yoga, is a style of yoga that was created by Bikram Choudhury during the 1970s. It is a particular succession of 26 stances and 2 breathing activities that are polished in a room warmed to 105°F (40.5°C) with a mugginess of 40%. The training is intended to expand strength, adaptability, and equilibrium, as well as advance by and large wellbeing and prosperity.

The 26 stances and 2 breathing activities are drilled in a similar request without fail, and are intended to work all aspects of the body efficiently. The succession starts with standing stances, including the Tree Posture and

Triangle Posture, and continues on toward situated stances, for example, the Bunny Posture and the Cobra Posture. The succession finishes up with the last stance, the Savasana, or Body Posture.

One of the vital elements of Bikram Yoga is the warmed room. The intensity and dampness help to heat up the muscles, increment adaptability, and advance detoxification by perspiring. The intensity additionally assists with working on cardiovascular wellbeing by expanding pulse and further developing blood stream to the muscles and organs.

One more significant part of Bikram Yoga is the accentuation on appropriate arrangement and structure. The succession of stances is intended to work each piece of the body with a certain goal in mind, and legitimate arrangement is fundamental to get the greatest advantage from each stance. Educators in Bikram Yoga are prepared to give explicit guidelines and acclimations to assist understudies with accomplishing appropriate arrangement and stay away from injury.

Bikram Yoga is a requesting practice, and isn't suggested for fledglings or those with wellbeing concerns. Notwithstanding, with standard practice and devotion, Bikram Yoga can assist with further developing strength, adaptability, and generally wellbeing and prosperity.

One of the critical advantages of rehearsing Bikram Yoga is worked on actual wellbeing. The training can assist with working on cardiovascular wellbeing, increment muscle strength and adaptability, and advance detoxification by perspiring. Customary practice can likewise assist with mitigating side effects of constant torment, like back agony and joint inflammation.

Notwithstanding the actual advantages, Bikram Yoga can likewise assist with working on psychological well-being and prosperity. The act of Bikram Yoga can assist with decreasing pressure and tension, further develop fixation and concentration, and advance sensations of serenity and inward harmony. Customary practice can likewise assist with further developing rest and increment energy levels.

Notwithstanding, there have been contentions encompassing Bikram Choudhury and his lessons, including claims of lewd behavior and wrongdoing. Subsequently, numerous yoga studios and experts have created some distance from the Bikram Yoga brand and have fostered their own styles of hot yoga.

All in all, Bikram Yoga is a particular succession of stances and breathing activities rehearsed in a warmed room. It is intended to expand strength, adaptability, and equilibrium, as well as advance generally wellbeing and prosperity. While it is a requesting practice, standard practice can assist with working on physical and emotional wellness, and advance a feeling of inward quiet and tranquility. Notwithstanding, it is vital to rehearse with alert and pay attention to your body, and to be aware of any discussions encompassing the Bikram Yoga brand.

Kundalini Yoga

Kundalini Yoga is a kind of yoga that spotlights on the enlivening of the Kundalini energy, which is supposed to be situated at the foundation of the spine. This training includes a mix of actual stances, breathing activities, contemplation, and reciting, and is intended to increment cognizance, bring issues to light, and advance profound development.

The term Kundalini is gotten from the Sanskrit word "kundal," and that signifies "snaked up." The Kundalini energy is in many cases depicted as a looped snake at the foundation of the spine, and the point of Kundalini Yoga is to stir this energy and move it up through the chakras, or energy focuses, of the body.

In Kundalini Yoga, the actual stances, or asanas, are utilized to set up the body for the enlivening of the Kundalini energy. These stances are in many cases dynamic and include tedious developments, for example, the "spinal flex," which includes on the other hand curving and adjusting the spine. The stances are intended to fortify the sensory system, increment adaptability, and further develop flow.

Breathing activities, or pranayama, are a significant part of Kundalini Yoga. These activities are utilized to actuate the Kundalini energy and move it up through the chakras. One of the most widely recognized breathing practices in Kundalini Yoga is the "breath of fire," which includes quick, musical breathing through the nose with equivalent accentuation on the breathe in and breathe out.

Reflection is likewise a critical part of Kundalini Yoga. This training includes zeroing in the brain on a solitary place of fixation, like the breath, a mantra, or a visual picture. In Kundalini Yoga, contemplation is frequently joined with the actual stances and breathing activities, and can be rehearsed in a situated or resting position.

Reciting, or mantra, is one more significant part of Kundalini Yoga. Mantras are hallowed sounds or expressions that are rehashed to assist with centering the brain and initiate the Kundalini energy. One of the most well-known mantras in Kundalini Yoga is "Sat Nam," and that signifies "truth is my personality."

A definitive objective of Kundalini Yoga is to stir the Kundalini energy and move it up through the chakras to the crown of the head, where it is said to join with the infinite cognizance. This enlivening is said to achieve a scope of advantages, including expanded mindfulness, elevated instinct, and a feeling of unity with the universe.

Kundalini Yoga is viewed as a strong practice, and moving toward it with watchfulness and respect is significant. It is suggested that amateurs practice under the direction of an accomplished instructor, and that people with specific ailments, for example, hypertension or epilepsy, talk with their primary care physician prior to starting the training.

Notwithstanding the profound advantages, Kundalini Yoga has been found to have a scope of physical and emotional well-being benefits. Studies have demonstrated the way that the training can assist with decreasing pressure and tension, work on resistant capability, and increment energy levels. It has likewise been viewed as powerful in the treatment of specific emotional well-being conditions, like gloom and habit.

All in all, Kundalini Yoga is a kind of yoga that spotlights on the enlivening of the Kundalini energy. It includes a blend of actual stances, breathing activities, contemplation, and reciting, and is intended to increment cognizance, bring issues to light, and advance otherworldly development. While it is viewed as a strong practice, it is critical to move toward it with watchfulness and regard, and to rehearse under the direction of an accomplished educator.

Yin Yoga

Yin Yoga is a style of yoga that includes holding latent, static postures for a few minutes all at once. Dissimilar to different sorts of yoga, which center around unique developments and stream, Yin Yoga stresses tranquility and unwinding.

The postures in Yin Yoga ordinarily focus on the connective tissues, like the tendons, ligaments, and belt, as opposed to the muscles. By holding the postures for longer timeframes, professionals can build their adaptability, scope of movement, and joint versatility.

Yin Yoga is likewise accepted to have remedial advantages for the body and brain. By holding the postures for expanded periods, specialists can animate the progression of energy or "qi" in the body, discharge pressure and stress, and work on mental clearness and concentration.

A few normal postures in Yin Yoga incorporate the butterfly present, mythical beast posture, and pigeon present. Props, for example, blocks and covers might be utilized to assist with supporting the body in the stances.

Yin Yoga can be drilled by individuals of all levels and capacities, and it very well may be an especially helpful practice for competitors or anybody hoping to work on their adaptability and portability. It is likewise a decent supplement to additional powerful styles of yoga or other proactive tasks, like running or weightlifting.

Restorative Yoga

Helpful yoga is a delicate and remedial style of yoga that spotlights on unwinding and stress decrease. It includes holding steady, serene postures for expanded timeframes, regularly 5-20 minutes or more, with the utilization of props like supports, covers, and blocks.

The motivation behind supportive yoga is to make a condition of profound unwinding in the body and brain, considering physical, mental, and close to home delivery. The long holds in the postures empower the body's unwinding reaction, diminishing pressure and tension, bringing down pulse, and advancing relaxing rest.

Helpful yoga is especially gainful for those recuperating from injury or disease, or those encountering persistent torment or stress. It can likewise be useful for those trying to adjust a more dynamic or energetic yoga practice.

A few normal helpful stances incorporate upheld youngster's posture, upheld span present, and leaned back bound point present. The utilization of props is fundamental in supportive yoga, as they help to make a feeling of solace and simplicity in the body, considering a more profound condition of unwinding.

Supportive yoga can be drilled by individuals of all levels and capacities, and it is many times prescribed as a corresponding practice to different types of activity, like running, weightlifting, or other more energetic styles of yoga.

The end.